I0410157

Eat! People Are Starving In Africa!

RV Siegel

EAT! PEOPLE ARE STARVING IN AFRICA!

100% of the profits of this book will be
donated to
<u>Stand Up For Kids Charity</u>

Providing hope and safe haven for the
street kids and
homeless children in America...

[www.standupforkids.org].

In this very personal yet scientifically accurate book, RV Siegel shares with her readers, one child's bad experiences with food. She was herself that child.

As a young girl, the author was taught that she always had to eat everything on her plate, even if she was not hungry. "There are children starving in Africa!" her mother would admonish. With a mixture of guilt and fear the child kept eating until eventually she had developed a serious weight problem. That was followed in adolescence by bouts of binging and purging, potentially fatal actions that she took not knowing what else to do.

Thankfully, RV Siegel was able to overcome what she came to call her "demon" and go on to live a normal life as an adult. But her own experiences led her to further research and the realization that poor eating habits - often so severe as to be life-threatening - have become an epidemic amongst millions of our children. Citing the latest research, this gripping book paints a starkly realistic portrayal of this grave problem…and what we as parents, educators and society at large can do to solve it!

To the children of this generation and for

the

generations to come you

are never alone.

For yesterday is but a dream

And tomorrow is only a vision…

But today, well-lived

Makes every yesterday a dream of happiness

And every tomorrow, a vision of Hope.

From: The Sanskrit

Acknowledgements

My love and thanks to Barry, David, and Amanda.

Table of Contents

EAT! PEOPLE ARE STARVING IN AFRICA!

BY

RV SIEGEL

* * * * * *

Success in weight loss among children and adolescents are short term. Our children will possibly be outlived by their parents because of obesity. Where and what are we heading for? Are these children haunted by the same demon? Must we start closer to home and see?

* * * * * *

PART ONE

My Crazy Life and I

"Eat! People are starving in Africa!"

It was thirty years ago, so I can't really tell if that was true or not. It just so happened that my grandmother and mother seemed to share this same global knowledge: People living in exotic parts of the world were somehow starving to death.

I was young and what did I know? So probably, that was true. Who could dare challenge that age-old (and possibly tested) wisdom?

My folks always admired "healthy looking" and "solid" kids. I remember Mother's rapturous encouragements, her face radiant with pride, whenever our plates were polished clean after a meal. In contrast, those foreboding dark brown eyes would be full of disappointment (and don't forget the wooden spoon!) if we said that we were not *that* hungry.

Eat! People Are Starving In Africa!

True enough, my mother could not see us healthy unless she packed our bones with "meat."

Somehow ingenious, although totally not recommended, she acquired some well-meaning advice from a few neighbors, and they too, believed that we needed some type of "vitamin" to help us "get bigger."

Mother determined that we did need more growing up (vertical or horizontal), to do.

She was advised that certain pills could just do that.

So off she went to the local pharmacy, where you could happily obtain prescription drugs without, a prescription from your physician.

I did not know exactly for how long, but I remember Celestone and Periactine were part of our daily "vitamin regimen," together with Flintstones MVI, Enervone-C and Trop-Iron (uh-huh, my mom decided we were also anemic – the cheeks were not rosy enough).

During mealtimes, mother thought of another creative way to make sure we ate fast enough. She would play Elvis Presley's LP album back to back. We had to finish the meal by the time the album got over.

Days went by. If I had a diary, this is what my entry would probably be:

Me at around age 4 years:

Day 1: Mommy gave us new vitamins today, yuck! I don't like those vitamins. Mommy said, "You should at least look like our cousins next door. They're a lot healthier". This afternoon, she was angry with me. She gave me the wooden spoon. Elvis Presley's LP album was over and I was still trying to finish my lunch. My sister Ella & brother Monty finished theirs much earlier (I will not tell mother that they gave their food to Wackie – the dog).

Day 3: Mommy said I was playing with my food. Not really. I was just scattering it around the plate so it would look like I was done. She said, God would punish me if I did that again and that I would go hungry – like those people in Africa (sometimes she used China).

Day 4: Ella threw up her supper while we were eating tonight. Mom was upset and my dad said to leave it alone. Monty and I finished supper quietly. I felt like gagging. Mom put so much food on our plates and it was difficult to finish it. I had to drink Ovaltine before bedtime too! Ooohhh, I have tummy ache. Ella's so lucky, she gets to sleep without finishing her plate.

Day 6: Mom found out about Wackie. Ella and Monty got the wooden spoon. My sister Ella was upset at mom too, she talked back to her. She said my mom was "not a good mother." Mom took some fish bones and shoved them inside Ella's mouth until it bled. I was really afraid. I will never talk back to mom --- ever. I'll be good and I'll take my vitamins.

Day 10: I finished my plate today! It was not hard at all. Mom said I was a good girl.

Eat! People Are Starving In Africa!

Day 14: Breakfast and lunch were great! I must have more snacks later in the day I am so hungry! I am always hungry. I'm tired too. I guess playing with my dolls does that. I'll just nap more. Mommy gets so happy when I nap in the afternoon. And oh boy, she gave me a great big hug and a bar of chocolate for being a good girl... I even finished my plate before Elvis Presley finished his last song from the LP album during suppertime! I'll do it again tomorrow. I'll be good.

Day 60: I am tired today. I'll play with my Chatty Cathy tomorrow. Mommy said Lola (grandmother) will be arriving from America after six sleeps. I wonder if naps count.

Finally at last! We grew and grew, side ways and up!

I learned years later that my mother, after almost a year of popping those "vitamins," thought something was awfully wrong with my sister, brother and I (she was eight, my brother was almost 6 and I was nearly 5 years old). For some reason, we seemed to develop "mumps" that would just not go away. It was later felt that these were the side effects of Celestone called "moon facies." A condition you acquire if you are a long-term user of steroid.

Me at almost 5 years:

Day 1: Mommy took the three of us to the Doctor. My little two years old brother Sunny stayed at home with the maid. Mommy said we didn't look right. I told her about my tummy aches too.

Day 2: Mommy told us that she would slowly start taking away the vitamins. After 10 sleeps, we wouldn't have to take any more vitamins except the Flintstones. I like that vitamin. Tastes like candy. I took two this morning. Mommy did not know.

Day 8: I am feeling tired and dizzy. I threw up. I'll write more stuff tomorrow.

Day 14: I did not go to school today. Mommy and daddy said I have allergies. My face is so swollen and my throat itches... heck, I itch all over. My doctor said I probably ate something that did not agree with me. I did not know food could agree or disagree… Can my food think? What's that suppose to mean? Can food get upset (like mommy) with me, too?

Day 55: I woke up in the school clinic. My teacher said daddy was coming over to pick me up, instead, Cita, our housemaid came to get me. We rode a taxi back home.

Day 60: It's been days and I still have not gone back to kindergarten. Mommy looks worried. It's my fault. I should have eaten all my breakfast and I should not have passed out again. Mom calls them "fits." I guess I am not healthy like my cousins, or Ella & Monty; I'll finish my plate from now on. I'll be good.

Day 61: The doctor told my mom that my white blood is more than my red blood. That's weird. I thought all blood was red! The nurse poked my finger and I screamed. It did not really hurt, but that should teach them not to poke me anymore.

Day 62: Ugh! I have to take all these yucky medicines. Mommy got mad when I spit out the thick medicine that's supposed to make my white blood red. My aunt arrived and I heard her talking to my mom. Mommy said the doctor thinks that I have leukemia but she was not really sure. Aren't doctors supposed to be powerful? Why does she have to ask my mommy to wait much longer? That's going to take forever! I am really sorry mommy. I am making her sadder with my fits.

Day 77: I cried all day today. The nurse poked my arm instead of my finger and it took three people to hold me down. I said 'No', but they still did it. Maybe God is really punishing me for stuff I did. I'm so tired. I'll start being good again after one nap. I don't know what made God angry though. Maybe Cita will tell me. Mommy is busy with Sunny (the baby).

Day 80: Mom made me eat that grilled liver... blood's still oozing from it, yuck! She said it's good for my condition – now that, I don't understand.

Eat! People Are Starving In Africa!

PS: Mommy stacked my plate with "Pinakbet" (Filipino cuisine made up of various vegetables). I told her I had finished my dinner and I threw it so Wackie could eat it.

Ok, those entries were really terrible. I cannot make it sound better. These were my memories as a child. almost of it seemed to surround issues like food, mealtimes, and my mother's obsession with making us "look healthy."

Obviously, my insecurities started to fester more and regrettably this was how my demon grew and intensified, haunting me for a long time.

About a year later, my family finally found out what was wrong with me. I was diagnosed with febrile seizures (it got resolved before I turned six), asthma, dermatographia, severe food allergy to shellfish and a benign type of childhood anemia for which I have no medical name since my mother cannot recollect that detail.

Eat! People Are Starving In Africa!

I guess, after a long-term use of steroids and antihistamines, being off those drugs finally triggered off all these illnesses. Truthfully, I may never know.

I started loathing vegetables since and it was not really hard to do.

"No more greens for me." There, I showed her!

Now, let us skip my uneventful childhood and travel through time: **My high-school years**. Sure, I spent 12 years in a private Catholic School and my four years in high school were very memorable indeed.

A diary? Oh yes, I tried those for a while back then. I've just had a hard time maintaining one since it seemed to be "just lying there" whenever my sister and mother were around.

You see, for me as a teenager, a diary was and still is as sacred as the Scriptures. It's where you pour your deepest thoughts and secrets, in short, your heart and soul – good or bad. I also used it to vent "negative feelings," whenever I harbored violent thoughts towards my siblings. Often, those thoughts played like a movie in my brain, especially after a routine quarrel with my brothers and sisters (particularly after being called "Miss Piggy" and "tabachoy" which is slang for 'very fat' in my native language).

I could not just yell and scream. I was the "good girl" and I would do anything not to mess that up.

In our household, talking back and being loud was a major taboo. You did not talk back, period. If my siblings poked fun at me, I was expected to practice the virtues of patience since I was an older child and could muster up the strength to resist immature behavior. For the record, four more siblings were born after Sunny, the fourth child (talking of which, eight is enough!).

"Pasensya ka na (let it go), you are older," Mother often yelled. "*And don't let me hear you talk back to Ella or Monty. They're older than you are.*"

Eat! People Are Starving In Africa!

Very soon after that, the banana trees planted in the backyard of the house became my best friends (although I do not think that those banana trees felt the same way) and convenient tools to help me vent my "feelings."

I screamed and yelled at them, punched and kicked them. Golly, even Wackie the dog can't take that!

Poor trees, that lot never bore any fruit thereafter.

Mother was baffled at this phenomenon. I heard her tell Cita that those banana trees were probably "male trees," therefore, would not bear fruit.

It was then, that I thought a diary would be a lot better.

I guess I have to add that to my guilty conscience --- I made those banana trees infertile!

Eat! People Are Starving In Africa!

So you see, I would have loved a diary to write all this stuff. However, I decided at that time that my thoughts were mine and mine alone. Again, if I had a diary, these would probably be my entries:

Freshman Years

Day 1: I'm in high school, at last! I can't believe it. Two more years and I'll get to attend a Prom. I am never allowed to go out with my friends to parties. I go to children's parties only to baby-sit my little brothers and sisters. Mom and dad were fighting again. The kids went to bed crying. Ella is having a meltdown. She turned off the light in the bedroom way before I got ready for bed. I'm here in the kitchen munching leftovers for supper. I'm not really hungry. It's like my stomach is full but my mouth wants more food. Mom told me tonight that she's glad that I'm around. I am the "responsible one" and "the strongest." I'm not really sure what she meant by that, but whatever it is, it sure made her smile.

Day 22: Next month is my birthday. I hope they won't forget it. Mom always cooks "pancit" and "adobo." Hmmm… I am hungry though. I wonder what we have in the refrigerator. I'll go see.

Day 27: Daniel smiled at me this morning. I love him so! I heard that he and Emmy are going out. Emmy told me they're "just friends". Emmy's been a good friend since 6th grade. She won't lie to me.

Day 38: Oh dear, my school uniform is getting tighter. I asked mom if I'm getting fat; she told me that I just looked "round." She also said that I should be thankful that I don't look like the children on the roads. Well, I still need to do something about my uniform. This weekend, I'll ask mom if I could get two new pairs. That'll be my birthday gift.

Day 45: I had a good day today. Mom did not forget my birthday and she cooked chicken, pancit, pork adobo, and we had ice cream. I think, I ate too much today. Ugh! I hate myself. Tomorrow, I'll go on a diet.

*Names mentioned in the "diary" had been modified.

Eat! People Are Starving In Africa!

Day 50: Darn it! All I think about today is food. I've been planning what and how much I should be eating since breakfast. I just raided the freezer and ate some more ice cream tonight. I finished the whole tub! Mom will be upset with me when she wakes up tomorrow.

Day 90: I'm officially 155 pounds now! Ella is only 95 pounds! Oh God, help me. I cannot stop.

Day 115: I'm so sick today. Mom said it could be food poisoning. I ate too many fish balls in school this afternoon. I'll probably stay home.

Day 116: Hey, I weighed myself this morning --- guess what? I am down to 150 pounds! Just for a day! Five whopping pounds off. I will definitely stop eating too much from now on. This is a good time to start dieting. Who knows, I may start looking like those models in the magazines. Listen up world: I'll finally be thin!!!

Day 120: What's happening to me? I weigh 157 pounds! I did not eat more than usual. Got to figure this out.

Day 127: Daniel told Emmy that it's impossible for him to even consider "liking" me. I was as fat as a pig! I can't believe Emmy told him. I cannot even look at both of them. After supper, Sunny and I had a fight. He called me a 'swine' and 'Miss Piggy' so I punched him. I hate myself. God help me!

Day 129: I keep opening the refrigerator door for no apparent reason. I just gaze at its contents and close the door. Later, I end up picking on leftovers. I'm not even hungry!

Day 133: I can just grab this flab all over me. I read somewhere that, if you could pinch over two inches of fat from your stomach and thighs, you were definitely FAT. Yes, that's me!

Eat! People Are Starving In Africa!

Day 138: I can't look at the mirror. All I see is a huge fat face. My face is so round. Hey you, Fatso --- yeah, you in the mirror. You need to lose weight. You look like a cow!

Day 155: I had to stop and sit for a while during PE. I feel so short of breath. Hmmm, maybe my asthma is acting up.

Day 180: Helloooo there….!!! I've done it. I've done it… Finally! It was not hard. All you have to do is to stick your finger and tickle your throat until you gag and throw up. I'll just do this for a while until I start losing weight. I'll know when to stop. No one will know.

Sophomore Years

Day 12: Guess what? My uniform still fits! I skipped lunch in school and ate very little tonight. Mom was too busy putting the little ones to sleep to notice.

Eat! People Are Starving In Africa!

Day 15: Darn it! I ate two hamburgers at lunch. The girls' restroom was full of kids so I didn't do my thing. Got to keep a look out. I skipped dinner tonight. Tomorrow, I'll skip breakfast and lunch. I'll make sure mom won't notice.

Day 29: I'm now down to 148 pounds. My uniform is becoming loose and my clothes are fitting a lot better. This is great. Maybe, Daniel will notice me, like Emmy (she's got a model's figure!). Anyway, my parents are still fighting. I've got to make peace here. School is good.

Day 57: Easy! I just thought about it, retch a little, and I throw up a lot. I don't even have to tickle my throat anymore. I think I deserve a chocolate pie. I'm down to 144 pounds!

Day 133: My throat hurts today. I threw up in the school bathroom this morning and I saw a little bit of blood. That's scary... I should lie low for now. I'll just have to watch my diet a little bit more. I wonder what those water pills do. I'll check it out

Eat! People Are Starving In Africa!

at the library and look up the pharmacy too. Ugh! I can still grab all this fat from my sides and tummy. I am soooo fat!

Yes, those were the days. I continued this habit through the rest of my high school and college years. I binged and self-induced vomit, or binged and skipped meals, and sometimes purged too. I had become so good at it that it was no sweat at all.

I have not vomited blood since that day though. I was glad. It scared me for a while and yet, the longing to be thin and be accepted by my peers was stronger. Nothing else was important. Nothing.

PART TWO

Coming Home To Self

The large and looming demon followed me everywhere in America. It was my own little secret and no one would know. I was more concerned about passing my State Board exam and practicing as a licensed Registered Nurse. Hopefully, I would be able to send enough money back home. My parents finally separated after I finished high school.

I passed the NCLEX exam and practiced as an RN concentrating on my first love --- Pediatrics. The more I worked, the more I learned about nursing, culture and diversity in USA.

In between my binges and self-induced vomiting, I decided to pursue higher education. I enrolled in a Masters program in Nursing at the local university where I met my future husband. I never told him about my demon. Right now, if I am careful, I'll stay put at 120-pounds. I stand 5 feet and 5 inches tall, and my weight is ideal vis a vis my height. And yet ----

Eat! People Are Starving In Africa!

The mirror tells me that I look alright. My clothes fit fine and I am a size six. Why do I still *feel fat?* Ok no one will know. I don't do *that* thing often anymore. Its just when I feel I overate, that's all.

Two years after my wedding and I got pregnant. My husband was ecstatic. I too, was very happy till I realized I *would get fat again.*

I thought about this at great length and then I decided. The demon would stay in me but he would not touch my unborn child.

****

Indeed, the demon stayed inside me. I could hear him taunt me in my subconscious mind. Somehow, the voice now seemed more an echo than a scream. Now, I was able to reconcile myself to the situation. I realized soon that the prevalent trend of obesity in this country was at a staggering all time high.

****

*Names mentioned in the "diary" had been modified.

Eat! People Are Starving In Africa!

I've interviewed various individuals, from families and friends, to old and new acquaintances, and even parents of my patients. I worked briefly as a Pediatric Nurse Practitioner specializing in Gastroenterology and Nutrition, and the Physician I worked with was an outstanding Pediatric Gastroenterologist in Boca Raton, Florida. I was amazed at the results of my findings. Parents' obsession with food and feeding their young appeared to be universal regardless of culture and ethnic backgrounds.

The US alone has spent over 40 billon dollars to fight obesity and yet, we are still losing the battle.

Success in weight loss among children and adolescents are short term. Our children will possibly be outlived by their parents because of obesity. Where and what are we heading for? Are these children haunted by the same demon? Must we start closer to home and see?

True, genetic factors and certain endocrinological problems contribute to obesity. But what about healthy children? Are we setting them up for failure at an early age?

Eat! People Are Starving In Africa!

The Research

I have not included this portion to simply sound scholarly, nor do I consider myself to be an expert.

Parental Perception of Childhood Obesity

Introduction

The prevention of child and adolescent obesity should be made a high priority. In 1998, the World Health Organization identified childhood obesity as a global epidemic [7, 25]. The fact that a large section of the population continues to suffer disproportionate levels of health problems, specifically childhood obesity, is still a major concern. Medical practitioners frequently encounter overweight children, and it would seem that current measures to prevent the problem have been unsuccessful, since related studies show the percentage of overweight children as a proportion of the population is continuing to rise.

According to Edward Sondik (2004), Director of the National Centers for Health Statistics (NCHS), one of the Centers for Disease Control and Prevention's (CDC's) National Center for Health

Statistics, the proportion of overweight children and adolescents, aged six to nineteen years of age has increased, from an average of 11% in 1988 to a staggering 15% between 1999 and 2000.

Further studies indicate that children who are overweight in the transition period face an increased risk of being overweight at seven years of age [31].

Consequences of Obesity in Children

Certain multi-system physiologic responses have also been shown to be associated with childhood obesity. According to the American Diabetes Association, (2000; 2004), these include hypertension, sleep apnea, insulin resistance, and pre-diabetes conditions such as impaired Glucose tolerance, impaired fasting glucose, and type- 2 diabetes. Birch and Fisher (1998; 1999) also suggest that aberrant behaviors may result from obesity in childhood. Further, research undertaken by Strauss (2000) correlates childhood obesity with low self-esteem, increased sadness, loneliness, and nervousness, which in turn results in the development of eating disorders and risky behaviors, such as smoking or excessive alcohol consumption.

Childhood obesity affects relationships with peers, increases stigmatization and social isolation, and can lead to a possible deterioration in the quality of family relationships [18]. Overweight individuals are more susceptible to a variety of negative conditions, including diabetes, cardiovascular disease, stroke, osteoarthritis, and certain cancers. Therefore, it is important to try and prevent childhood obesity, particularly early in life, in order to reduce the dramatic overall upward trend in the prevalence of obesity.

Parents, the Family and Childhood Obesity

Parental perception and their understanding of childhood obesity play a prominent role in influencing their attitudes about childhood feeding and childhood feeding control [9]. These perceptions not only affect parenting styles with regard to appropriation of food, but also the child's health and the overall nutritional value of their diet. Hodges (2003) explores the influence of parenting styles, parental eating patterns, environment, and genetics as precursors to weight problems and obesity in children.

Clear communication, adequate behavioral control and structured planning within families helps promote healthy behavior in children; and this extends to nutrition [7]. In addition, researchers also have explored the phenomena that surrounds controlled child-feeding practices [3, 10, 26].

Prevalence and Trends of Obesity Among Children and Adolescents

A survey on the prevalence and trends of obesity among children and adolescents (six to 17 years old) in the United States was conducted by The National Health Examination Survey (NHES) II & III, and the National Health and Nutrition Examination Surveys (NHANES) from 1963 through 1994 and the NHANES I, 1971 to 1974; NHANES II, 1976 to 1980; and NHANES III, 1988 to 1994 respectively. The survey took into account this section of the population with respect to sex, age, race/ethnicity, income, and educational levels. Prevalence of obesity increased over time, with the highest point being touched between the NHANES II & III cycles.

What is Childhood Obesity?

The amount of research related to childhood obesity has increased in the past 40 years. Part of the issues that came forth was the struggle to obtain a correct definition of obesity among children and adolescents.

Before we define obesity empirically it is necessary to be acquainted with the different measures of obesity.

Measures of obesity:

A review of related articles indicated various means proposed by experts, on how to measure obesity among children and adolescents. These are however, not limited to the following:

1. Measurements based on adiposity (or 'fatness').
2. Measures of weight and height as well as of thickness of the skinfold from several anatomic sites.
3. The use of body mass index (BMI; kg/M2).
4. Combination of BMI (body mass index) and adiposity in youth while considering other factors such as gender, race, age, and status of maturation.
5. The use of a well-known statistical criterion like the growth charts to characterize the full distribution of measurement (height, weight) or measurement ratio (weight-for-height, BMI) across ages for children.

Often, in epidemiologic applications, growth charts can form the basis for evaluation of a cross-section of data by becoming a reference point from which a particular percentile cutoff is chosen to classify individuals as overweight, underweight, stunted, etc. [15].

Empirical (Measurable) Definition of Obesity in Children:

Being overweight was defined by age and a sex specific 95th percentile of body mass index (BMI) from NHES II & III (cycle II, 1963 to 1965; Cycle III, 1966 to 1970) and the NHANES I, II, & III. BMI values between the 85th and 95 percentiles were considered as the areas of concern, because in these levels, there was increased possibility for becoming obese [38].

In the past 30 years, researchers and experts have generally agreed that the 95th percentile of BMI is used to define the phenomena of being overweight. These criteria are most likely to be specific for obesity than lower percentile cutoffs. The 85th percentile has been used to classify adults as overweight, and between the 85th

*Names mentioned in the "diary" had been modified.

and 95th percentile cutoffs are those who are at risk for becoming overweight eventually.

What do parents think about obesity?

To date, although thousands of articles related to childhood obesity are readily available, research on parental perceptions of childhood obesity and nutrition remain scarce. A research study in 1980 explored parental perceptions of their children's body sizes. Interestingly, this study revealed that mothers served their overweight sons far larger portions of food compared to their non-overweight brothers. Perhaps the perception here was that they were bigger boys and therefore, needed more food [40].

Another provocative data surfaced regarding perception of children's growth. It pointed to the fact that the child's place on the growth curve was directly related to his or her health and parenting competence. In short, the higher the child was on the growth curve, the healthier it was and the more competent the parents proved [2]. Similar studies also showed congruencies in parental perceptions of their obese children: they fell short of recognizing their children as obese despite the empirical measurements [2, 17, 32].

Surprisingly, the children were not believed to be overweight if they were active and had a healthy diet and/or a good appetite [17]. Overweight children were described as thick or solid. Mothers believe that an inherited tendency to become overweight was likely to be in the child regardless of environmental factors [17].

Introduction of non milk foods for infants

Maternal perception of an infant's body size was positively correlated with the early introduction of nonmilk foods. Significantly, more infants perceived as small were introduced to nonmilk foods earlier, compared to infants who were perceived as average. Also, in the same study, infants who were introduced earlier to nonmilk foods had a greater infant BMI at six -7 months of age [4].

Eat! People Are Starving In Africa!

What Does It Mean?

Data analysis revealed that lack of parental control and unrestricted eating; increased parental control or application of dietary restrictions; their knowledge of nutrition; perceptions of self; and of childhood obesity were the predominant categorical antecedents of parental perceptions of obesity in their children.

Lack of parental control and unrestricted eating were described as lack of control over the family diet. Furthermore, it was described as a feeling of powerlessness to remedy the situation or just simply unwillingness to make changes.

Another dimension that is noteworthy is the inability to say 'no' if the child claimed to be hungry. Withholding food would mean starving the child. The inability to limit the child's eating also suggests that parents used food as a parenting tool or to reward children. Reluctance to limit or to withhold certain foods also indicated certain association with pride of being able to provide "treats" and has been a phenomenon in itself. This occurrence was strongly reported by low-income mothers in the Jain, et al. (2001) qualitative study.

Increased parental control over children's intakes revealed several provocative propositions with regard to parental perceptions of childhood obesity. Heavier parents dominated increased reports of restriction over food with heavier children [11]. Again, in lieu of the application of discipline, parents described withholding palatable "bad" foods as a form of punishment. Indeed, parents spontaneously reported the belief that restricting or forbidding the consumption of a particular food would decrease their child's preference for that food [6], a prediction contrary to research findings [3].

The child's eating styles also appeared to prompt concern and control over feeding. This elicited fear and distress that their child was at risk of obesity [34].

Interestingly, research indicates that obese individuals eat at a faster rate than non-obese persons [34]. It also proposes that the degree of maternal control correlates with maternal self-perception of who is overweight and obese.

Parental knowledge of nutrition suggests that it goes hand in hand with their readiness to learn and understand the concepts of nutrition and health, particularly with their children [13, 19].

Parental Perception: Children's Body Sizes, Food Choices and Activities

Parental perceptions of childhood obesity, has included descriptions like 'being big-boned' or 'having a large frame'. This is culturally acceptable and even desirable. Mothers verbalized no concern over body size and weight until the child's clothing had to be purchased too frequently indicating rapid growth [17].

Concerns were raised by parents regarding the child's size if the child became inactive or was being teased by peers due to his or her obesity. It was also strongly suggested that being overweight caused inactivity rather than the other way around [17].

*Names mentioned in the "diary" had been modified.

Moreover, mothers described obesity as a condition that caused severe functional impairments. Food intake was not much of a concern as long as the child ate certain foods such as fruits and vegetables. Parents believed that eating fruits and vegetables resulted in a healthy diet and the child was then considered healthy regardless of the amount and nutritional quality of other foods in the diet. It was implied that the intake of fruits and vegetables (as healthy foods) compensated for eating junk foods [17].

Children and the Growth Charts as Perceived by Parents

There is a strong positive correlation of perceived maternal competence and the position of their child on the growth chart [2]. The higher the child is plotted on the curve of the growth chart, the better parenting skills the mother has.

Attributes

Identification and analysis of the attributes of Parental Perception on Childhood Obesity yielded seven categories or dimensions to the concept. First was the maternal self-perception of obesity. Characteristics of this dimension included parents' reports of obesity and its status. Studies indicated that parents (mothers) who were overweight or obese were able to report their measured weight with high correlation of their self-perceived body weight (estimation of weight) and body size accurately.

Second, was parental influence that included the exercise of parenting skills, styles, and eating patterns, division of responsibility between parents and child, and application of behavior control.

Third, were the familial attributes. Exemplary characteristics were the role of family functions and genetics in the development of obesity in children. Also included here were inherent characteristics such as gender, age, and ethnicity.

Fourth, was the socio-environmental dimension that included the physical environment of the child and his or her family, societal values, socio-economic status, education, communication and language.

Fifth, was the psychological category that resulted in the development of obesity during childhood. These categories were low self-esteem, loneliness, isolation, poor peer and familial relationship, and the possible development of eating disorders and / or aberrant behaviors.

Sixth, was the parental food / nutrition competency. This attribute was characterized by comprehension of food labels and nutrition knowledge.

Consequences

Identification and analysis of the consequences of Parental Perceptions of Childhood Obesity yielded four major categories but were not limited to the following:

1. Increased prevalence of obesity.
2. Decreased self-esteem.
3. Development of obesity-related illnesses.
4. Children's inability to regulate food consumption.

Surrogate and Related Terms

Multidisciplinary studies used similar surrogate and related terms in expressing childhood obesity. Overweight and obesity were terms used interchangeably across the disciplines. One author described obesity as the "socially constructed phenomena and has inherent psychosocial implications and psychological meaning for individual" [12], while other authors stated that "childhood obesity can be viewed as not being able to keep oneself in balance and harmony in a complex existence between the child's physical and psychological health, and his or her interactions with the family and society" [7]. Intriguingly, many laypersons described obesity among children as simply as them being "thick or solid," "big-boned," and "large framed" [17, 40].

Theoretical Framework

Theoretical frameworks are tools used by researchers in an effort to describe, predict, or explain an observable fact, occurrence, or phenomena.

1. The concept of cognitive behavioral theory under which the cognitive-behavioral modification interventions can be used for problem solving, goal setting, self-monitoring, cognitive restructuring, and behavior modification to control eating and activity behaviors [1].

2. The social learning theory strengthened behavioral intervention by the use of reinforcement and punishment and modeling to control/change behavior [1].

3. The social influences theory, which was used as a model for Healthy for Life (H. F. L.) program design. It proposed that adolescent health behaviors and decisions were based primarily on the social meaning perceived in a specific social setting [24].

4. The Piagetian theory proposed that children between two to seven years of age were in the pre-operational stage [35]. During this period (which has two substages), intelligence was demonstrated through the use of symbols. Language use, memory and imagination are developed too. However, thinking is done in a non-logical, non-reversible manner. Egocentric thinking predominates [15]. It is believed that the child between two and seven years learns by manipulating his or her environment rather than by passive listening [39]. According to this theory, nutrition and education for this age group should involve activity-based teaching and teaching strategies, which encourage interaction with the real world (i.e., food). They (parents) need to find ways to teach abstract concepts, as

nutrients in meaningful ways. This must be clearly understood to impact these children's food choices.

5. The Family Collaborative Ecosystemic Model (FEM), developed by Goetz and Caron in 1999 is also a sound theory model [7]. It suggests that there is a significant relationship between health behaviors of the child and his or her family, implying that the environment is an important part of the child's health status and behavior.

6. Another potential framework [16] for prevention of obesity in children is the Satter's (1996) Trust Model. It proposes that health care providers and parents should rely on what she (Satter) refers to as "trust" paradigm instead of the current "control" paradigm for understanding childhood obesity. In this theory, it is believed that infants and young children have the ability to determine their own internal cues of hunger and satiety [3, 29,30].

Summary of the Study Findings

Over all, the findings indicate multi disciplinary consensus on the antecedents, attributes, and consequences of parental perception of childhood obesity. Furthermore, the results propose that the antecedents of parental perceptions of childhood obesity cultivate the manifestation of the attributive dimensions of parental perception of childhood obesity. Several consequences flow from these dimensions. These consequences in turn, strengthen the antecedents and actualization of parental perceptions of childhood obesity, thereby reinforcing the cycle of concept development.

*Names mentioned in the "diary" had been modified.

Discussion

The present analysis, based on the data representing the phenomena, contributes to the enduring conceptual development of parental perceptions of childhood obesity. The present study implies that parental perceptions of childhood obesity have universally conflicting attributes, which make it more complex.

Further conceptual investigation on parental perceptions of childhood obesity is clearly indicated. It is essential to corroborate the global defining characteristics of parental perceptions of childhood obesity.

Current intervention studies that are based on multiple variables such as nutrition education, family, community (i.e. project Headstart, WIC), school, and clinical/primary care based interventions appear to be promising and should be supported by the public at large.

Findings suggest that more instrument development and psychometric research needs to be conducted with a variety of audiences, which should include culture and sensitivity to changing needs [8].

Further investigation is warranted with regard to: changes in eating behavior over time [20], exploration of a theoretical framework that is based on family theory [1], the relationship between social learning and food preferences and/or food acceptance patterns [35], and the relationship of parental influence with perception and its effects on the development of eating behaviors in children [3,11,16,17,33].

Aberrant psychological behavior may also result in conjunction with obesity. It was surmised that societal values equating physical attractiveness and fitness with femininity, fostered a pervasive trend of dieting in most young women, many of whom did not need to lose weight. Dietary restrictions involving cognitive restrictions on food intake that involved explicit denial of hunger cues caused one to stop eating while still hungry and skip meals [11].

Eat! People Are Starving In Africa!

The relationship between childhood obesity and low self-esteem also indicated positive correlations. Pervasiveness of increased rates of sadness, loneliness, and nervousness usually accompanied low self-esteem resulting from obesity, specifically during adolescence. This in turn resulted in aberrant and risky behaviors such as smoking tobacco or consuming alcohol [33].

The importance of consistent family support and intervention, levels of education and socio economic status [24], would most likely report positive outcomes, not only with risky behaviors, but also with obesity control and prevention.

In exploring eating behaviors among children, family structure, exercise, and behavioral interventions would most likely improve overall outcomes [1]. Food preferences or food acceptance patterns appeared to be linked with past experiences with food and social learning [35], thus strengthening the proposition that immediate environmental factors such as the family strongly influences children's behavior.

PART THREE

Let's Take The Reins

After observing a sliver of parental perceptions of childhood obesity, we have a much better understanding of how to objectively tackle this issue.

It took me years to attempt to understand and sort out personal and internal conflicts before I realized that there was hope in conquering what seemed to be a wild, uncontrolled behemoth.

Now, let's take control and arm ourselves with knowledge to fight our enemy, since we know how it operates.

Interpreting Anthropometric Data for Infants, Children and Adolescents

Ideal Weight for Height & Percent Ideal Weight for Height

Morrison & Hark's (1996) formula in obtaining ideal weight for height and percent ideal weight for height of a child has been utilized here. Most parents are familiar with the National Center for Health Statistics' (NCHS) Physical Growth Chart, or simply, the pink and blue growth charts that one sees in the Pediatrician's office.

Copies of these growth charts have been included at the end of this book, formatted to fit, so you can do these exercises at leisure. These charts can also be downloaded and printed from http://www.cdc.gov/nchs/about/major/nhanes/growthcharts/. Other reference material may be seen at http://www.cdc.gov/nccdphp/dnpa/bmi/ for more on BMI (Body Mass Index) for Children and Teens.

Now, the exercise:

1. Plot your child's actual height / length on the appropriate growth chart for his or her age.
2. Find the point where the height intersects the 50th percentile on the height/length chart by moving horizontally right or left.

3. Draw a line down from this intersection on the height chart to the X-axis to find the age that corresponds to this 50th percentile height.

4. Find and record the 50th percentile weight for that age on the weight chart. This is the ideal weight for the child's current height.

Example A: Bruce is a 25 months old baby boy (so you will use the MALE 0-36 months growth chart). His current height is 88.9 cm or 35 inches [50th percentile]. His current weight is 16.36 kg or 36 lbs. [over the 95th percentile mark]. Bruce's ideal weight for current height is 13 kg or 28.5 pounds.

This is how inches (in) convert to centimeters (cm):

Inches

$$\frac{\text{Inches}}{0.3937} = cm$$

>> Therefore: 35/0.3937 = 88.9 cm.

This is how pounds (lbs) convert to kilograms (kg):

$$\frac{pounds}{2.2} = kilograms\ (kg)$$

>>Therefore: 36/2.2 = 16.36 kg.

The percent ideal weight for height is a number used to determine the degree of wasting or obesity in children and adolescents. Percent ideal weight for height describes the extent of any related changes in body composition resulting from intake deficits. This value is calculated by dividing the current weight by ideal weight for height.

Thus:

$$Percent\ weight\ for\ height = \frac{current\ weight}{Ideal\ weight\ for\ current\ height} \times 100$$

Example B: In case of Bruce, we know that his ideal weight for current height is 13 kg or 28.5 lbs.

>>Therefore: $\dfrac{16.36 \text{ kg}}{13\text{kg}} \times 100 = 125.8$ or 126%

So Bruce's actual weight is 126% of his ideal weight based on his height, which leads to the diagnosis of obesity.

Interpretation of Percent Ideal Weight for Height According to Morrison & Hark (1996):

% WEIGHT FOR HEIGHT	INTERPRETATION
Over 120	Obese
110 – 120	Overweight
90-109	Normal Weight
80-89	Mild Wasting
70-79	Moderate Wasting
Less than 70	Severe wasting

BMI for Children and Teens

Another common method in assessing weight among children and teens is by the use of the body mass index (BMI). This tool is useful in evaluating whether the child is underweight, overweight, or at risk for obesity. It is known that fatness among children changes as they grow. Also, girls and boys differ in body sizes as they mature. This is why BMI for children, also referred to as **BMI-for-age**, is gender and age-specific. BMI-for-age is plotted on age specific growth charts. These charts are used for children and teens between the ages 2 and 20.

Each of the CDC (Center for Disease Control) BMI-for-age gender specific charts contains a series of curved lines indicating specific percentiles. Healthcare professionals use the following established percentile cut-off points to identify instances of children being underweight and overweight.

Underweight	BMI-for-age: less than 5th percentile.
At risk of overweight	BMI-for-age 85th percentile to less than 95th percentile
Overweight	BMI-for-age: over 95th percentile.

It is known that BMI decreases during the pre school years, then increases as the child proceeds into adulthood. The percentile curves show this pattern of growth.

What does it mean when my Practitioner says that my child is in the 75th percentile?

The 75th percentile means a lower BMI when compared to the children of the same gender and age.

Why is BMI-for-Age a useful tool?

BMI-for-Age is a useful tool because:

1. It provides a reference for adolescents that can be used beyond puberty.

2. Children and adolescents compare well to laboratory measures of body fat (high correlation).

3. It can be used to track body size throughout life.

Important Information:

BMI, specifically for adults is only a part of an overall diagnostic tool to determine risk factors for diseases and death. Two people can have the same BMI, but a different percent body fat. A body builder with a large muscle mass and a low percent body fat may have the same BMI as a person who has more body fat. This is because BMI is calculated using weight and height only.

To learn more about Adult BMI, please check the CDC's website at: http://www.cdc.gov/nccdphp/dnpa/bmi/bmi-adult.htm.

How to Calculate Your Own BMI (for mommies & daddies)

English Formula:

BMI = $\dfrac{\text{weight in pounds}}{(\text{Height in Inches}) \times (\text{Height in inches})}$ X 70

Metric Formula:

BMI= $\dfrac{\text{weight in kilograms}}{(\text{Height in meters}) \times (\text{height in meters})}$

BMI= $\dfrac{\text{weight in kilograms}}{(\text{Height in cm}) \times (\text{height in cm})}$ X 10,000

Eat! People Are Starving In Africa!

Note

If you decide to do the exercises above and it raises more questions than answers on your part, you are asked to speak to your Pediatrician or Nurse Practitioner as soon as possible. Certain underlying conditions and / or disorders such as malabsorption, endocrinological, etc. may be the culprits, which could definitely require further medical attention.

PART FOUR

Frequently Asked Questions

What is Celestone?

Celestone (generic = bethamethasone) is a synthethic, long-acting glucocorticoid with minor mineralocorticoid properties but strong immunosuppressive, antinflammatory, and metabolic action.

What is Periactine?

Periactine (generic = cyproheptadine hydrochloride) is a potent piperidine antihistamine. It produces mild central depression and moderate anticholinergic effects. It is also used as an appetite stimulant (unlabeled use).

Can I ask my Physician for Periactine for my child? Its said, its unlabeled use is as an appetite stimulant.

Sure, but also it must be understood that all medication have side effects. Even ones, which are over-the-counter. Close medical supervision is needed for any type of treatment, which includes administration of medications and even supplements. Your child's weight must also be monitored closely. For the prescription medication Periactine, its side effects stimulate the appetite while making you sleepy and tired.

How about herbal supplements?

I am very wary of herbal supplements. I will never recommend herbal supplements for children since there is no empirical study with regard to children and uses of herbs. Children absorb medications and chemicals very differently. That is why your Practitioner almost always determines your child's weight first before prescribing any type of drug. Besides, if you steep green tea for one minute vs. three minutes in a cup, how much is the actual quantity of this tea in the first cup vs. the second cup? Lastly, more and more research determines that certain herbal supplements you find over-the-counter may interact with your child's medications, at times, with a very grievous outcome.

Why is self-induced vomiting bad for us?

Vomiting not only causes your body to lose fluids, but also induces electrolyte imbalances. Vomiting may harm the lining of your esophagus (the tube where food passes from your mouth to stomach). Your stomach contains certain acids used by your body to breakdown food for digestion. Once these acids escape the stomach to travel back to the esophagus, in the long run, it will cause the cells on your esophagus to mutate or change. This is called Barrett's Esophagus, a precursor stage of esophageal cancer.

I think my child is making herself throw up, what should I do?

Get help. **NOW**. Even if you just suspect it. You must include your child's Primary Care Practitioner (PCP) in this challenge. It will take a multidisciplinary team in order to help your child. This may include a Gastroenterologist, Psychiatrist, Nutritionist, Dietician, etc. Whatever it takes, **YOU** and only you are the best advocate for this troubled teen. Take the rein and hang on. When in doubt, ask for a second opinion.

PART FIVE

In Closing...

The bottom line is *you are not alone*. Understanding different, possible factors that influence childhood obesity is the first step to facing up to this demon. In the hope that our personal demon does not affect our ways with our children by over-compensating on what we should and should not do (restrictions vs. over-indulgence of palatable foods), I feel that healthy children have their own "on and off" buttons that determine their satiety. We must be able to tune in to their subtle cues. They may be saying that they are satisfied and full, and yet, we are so occupied with that "one last ounce" left in the bottle or "just two more bites" on their plate that we are ignoring this innate determination of satiety.

As said before, I am not an expert. I am here to tell my story and what I ended up doing. I armed myself with knowledge so I could understand better. This is not the final battle. This is just the beginning.

---

*Names mentioned in the "diary" had been modified.

Eat! People Are Starving In Africa!

Sure, I still hate my vegetables, but children model themselves on their parents. If you think that "they don't know," please think again. Children are wonderfully blessed with intelligence that we seldom appreciate and often underestimate.

I believe utilizing the Food Pyramid is still a great start. I am a firm believer of calorie control. What you get depends on what and how much you eat. Discuss this with your healthcare providers and let them guide you in calculating calorie intake specific to your growing child.

The original "Four Food Groups" has been replaced with the "Food Guide Pyramid". This illustrates the relative proportions of different foods that make up a nutritious, well-balanced diet.

PART SIX

My Notes

Please use this portion of the book as a journal and jot some concerns and/or questions that you may have as you read this book.

Date	My Notes	Activities	Evaluation

Eat! People Are Starving In Africa!

Date	My Notes	Activities	Evaluation

Eat! People Are Starving In Africa!

Date	My Notes	Activities	Evaluation

Eat! People Are Starving In Africa!

Eat! People Are Starving In Africa!

MY NOTES

Eat! People Are Starving In Africa!

MY NOTES

Eat! People Are Starving In Africa!

MY NOTES

Eat! People Are Starving In Africa!

MY NOTES

Eat! People Are Starving In Africa!

Eat! People Are Starving In Africa!

Growth Charts: SET 1 - 10

*Names mentioned in the "diary" had been modified.

Birth to 36 months: Boys
Length-for-age and Weight-for-age percentiles

NAME _____

RECORD # _____

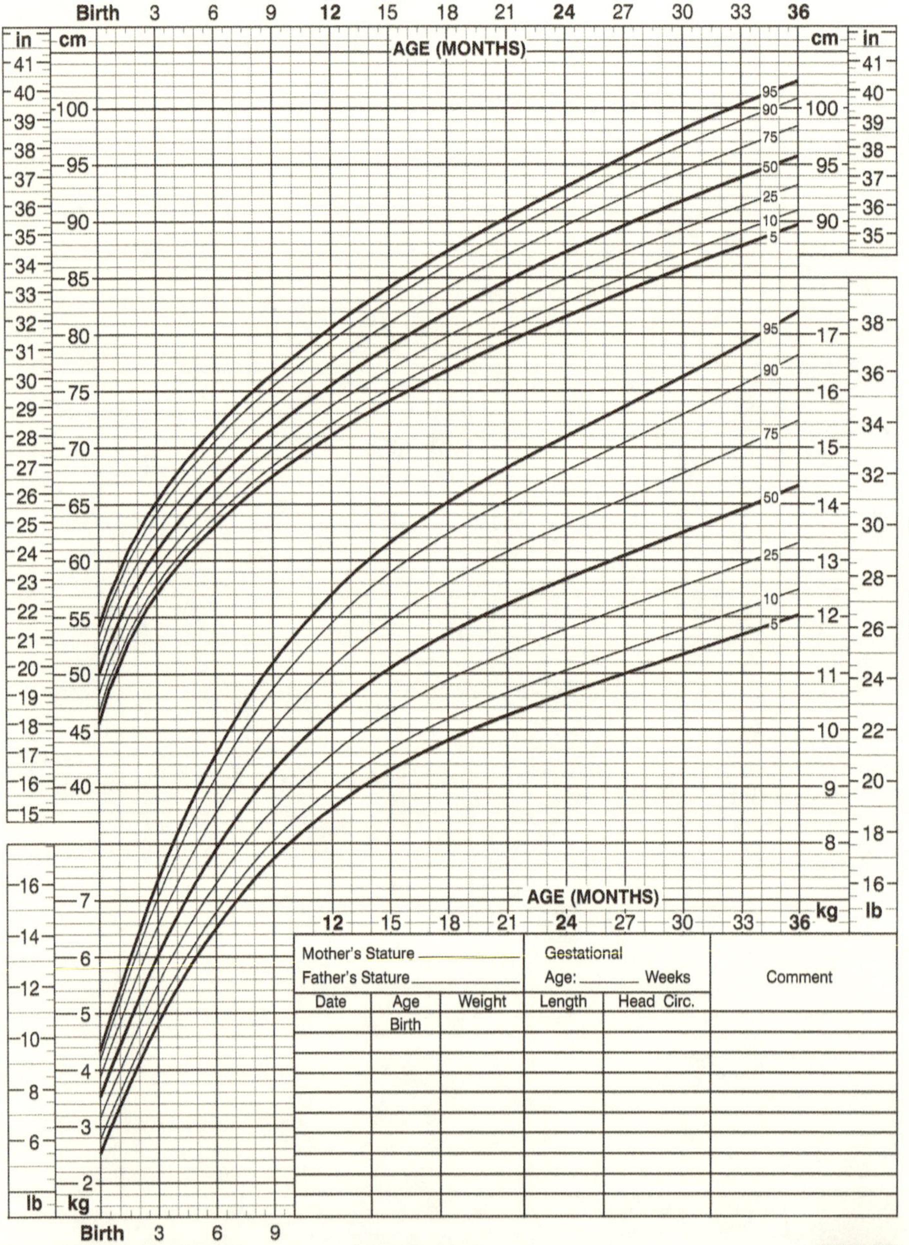

AGE (MONTHS)

Birth 3 6 9 12 15 18 21 24 27 30 33 36

LENGTH (in / cm)

Percentile curves labeled (upper/length): 95, 90, 75, 50, 25, 10, 5

WEIGHT (lb / kg)

Percentile curves labeled: 95, 90, 75, 50, 25, 10, 5

AGE (MONTHS)

12 15 18 21 24 27 30 33 36

		Gestational		Comment
Mother's Stature _____		Age: _____ Weeks		
Father's Stature _____				
Date	Age	Weight	Length	Head Circ.
Birth				

Birth 3 6 9

Published May 30, 2000 (modified 4/20/01).
SOURCE: Developed by the National Center for Health Statistics in collaboration with
the National Center for Chronic Disease Prevention and Health Promotion (2000).
http://www.cdc.gov/growthcharts

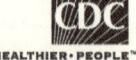

SAFER · HEALTHIER · PEOPLE™

Birth to 36 months: Girls
Length-for-age and Weight-for-age percentiles

NAME _____

RECORD # _____

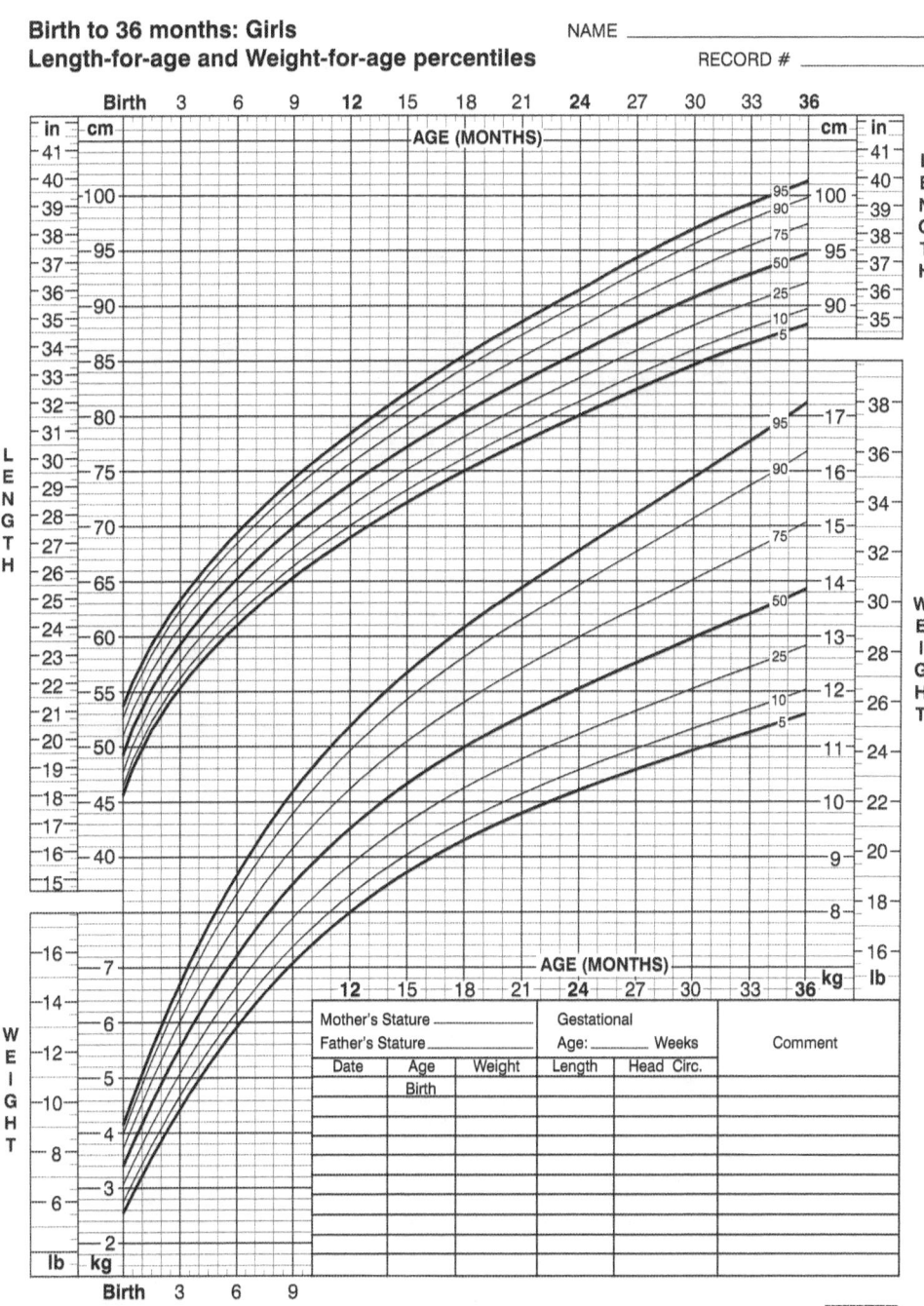

Mother's Stature _____
Father's Stature _____
Gestational Age: _____ Weeks

Date	Age	Weight	Length	Head Circ.	Comment
Birth					

Published May 30, 2000 (modified 4/20/01).
SOURCE: Developed by the National Center for Health Statistics in collaboration with
the National Center for Chronic Disease Prevention and Health Promotion (2000).
http://www.cdc.gov/growthcharts

CDC
SAFER · HEALTHIER · PEOPLE™

Birth to 36 months: Boys
Head circumference-for-age and
Weight-for-length percentiles

NAME _____

RECORD # _____

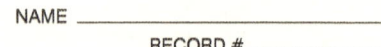

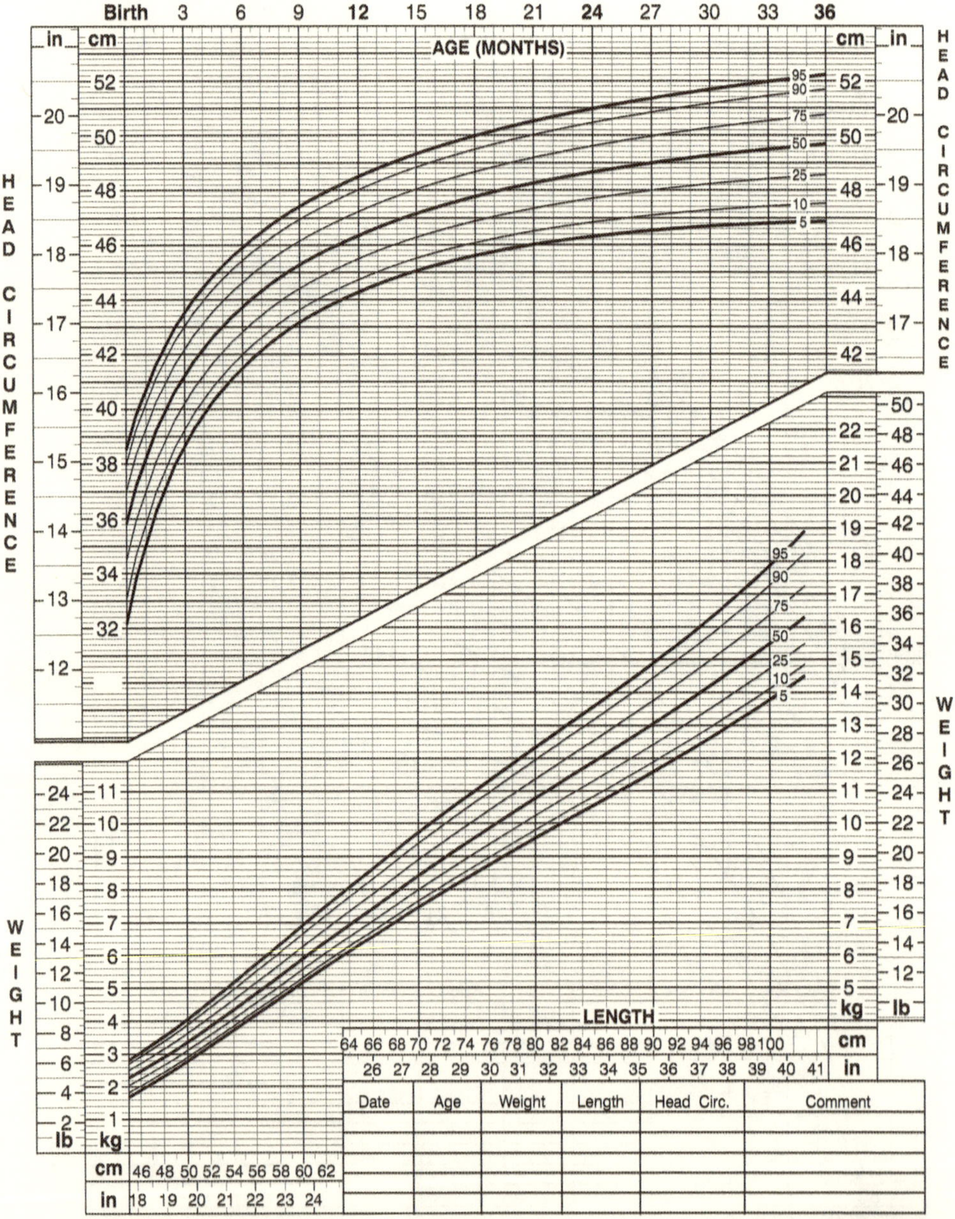

AGE (MONTHS)

Birth 3 6 9 12 15 18 21 24 27 30 33 36

HEAD CIRCUMFERENCE

in cm

52
50
48
46
44
42
40
38
36
34
32

20
19
18
17
16
15
14
13
12

95
90
75
50
25
10
5

WEIGHT

LENGTH

cm 64 66 68 70 72 74 76 78 80 82 84 86 88 90 92 94 96 98 100
in 26 27 28 29 30 31 32 33 34 35 36 37 38 39 40 41

kg lb

24 11
22 10
20 9
18 8
16 7
14 6
12 5
10 4
8 3
6
4 2
2 1
lb kg

cm 46 48 50 52 54 56 58 60 62
in 18 19 20 21 22 23 24

Date	Age	Weight	Length	Head Circ.	Comment

Published May 30, 2000 (modified 10/16/00).
SOURCE: Developed by the National Center for Health Statistics in collaboration with
the National Center for Chronic Disease Prevention and Health Promotion (2000).
http://www.cdc.gov/growthcharts

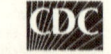

SAFER · HEALTHIER · PEOPLE™

Birth to 36 months: Girls
Head circumference-for-age and
Weight-for-length percentiles

NAME _____

RECORD # _____

AGE (MONTHS)

Birth 3 6 9 12 15 18 21 24 27 30 33 36

HEAD CIRCUMFERENCE

in — cm

52
20
50
19 — 48
18 — 46
44
17 — 42
16 — 40
15 — 38
14 — 36
34
13 — 32
12

95
90
75
50
25
10
5

HEAD CIRCUMFERENCE

WEIGHT

LENGTH

64 66 68 70 72 74 76 78 80 82 84 86 88 90 92 94 96 98 100 cm
26 27 28 29 30 31 32 33 34 35 36 37 38 39 40 41 in

Date	Age	Weight	Length	Head Circ.	Comment

cm 46 48 50 52 54 56 58 60 62
in 18 19 20 21 22 23 24

Published May 30, 2000 (modified 10/16/00).
SOURCE: Developed by the National Center for Health Statistics in collaboration with
the National Center for Chronic Disease Prevention and Health Promotion (2000).
http://www.cdc.gov/growthcharts

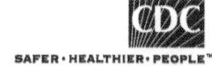

SAFER · HEALTHIER · PEOPLE™

2 to 20 years: Boys
Stature-for-age and Weight-for-age percentiles

NAME _____

RECORD # _____

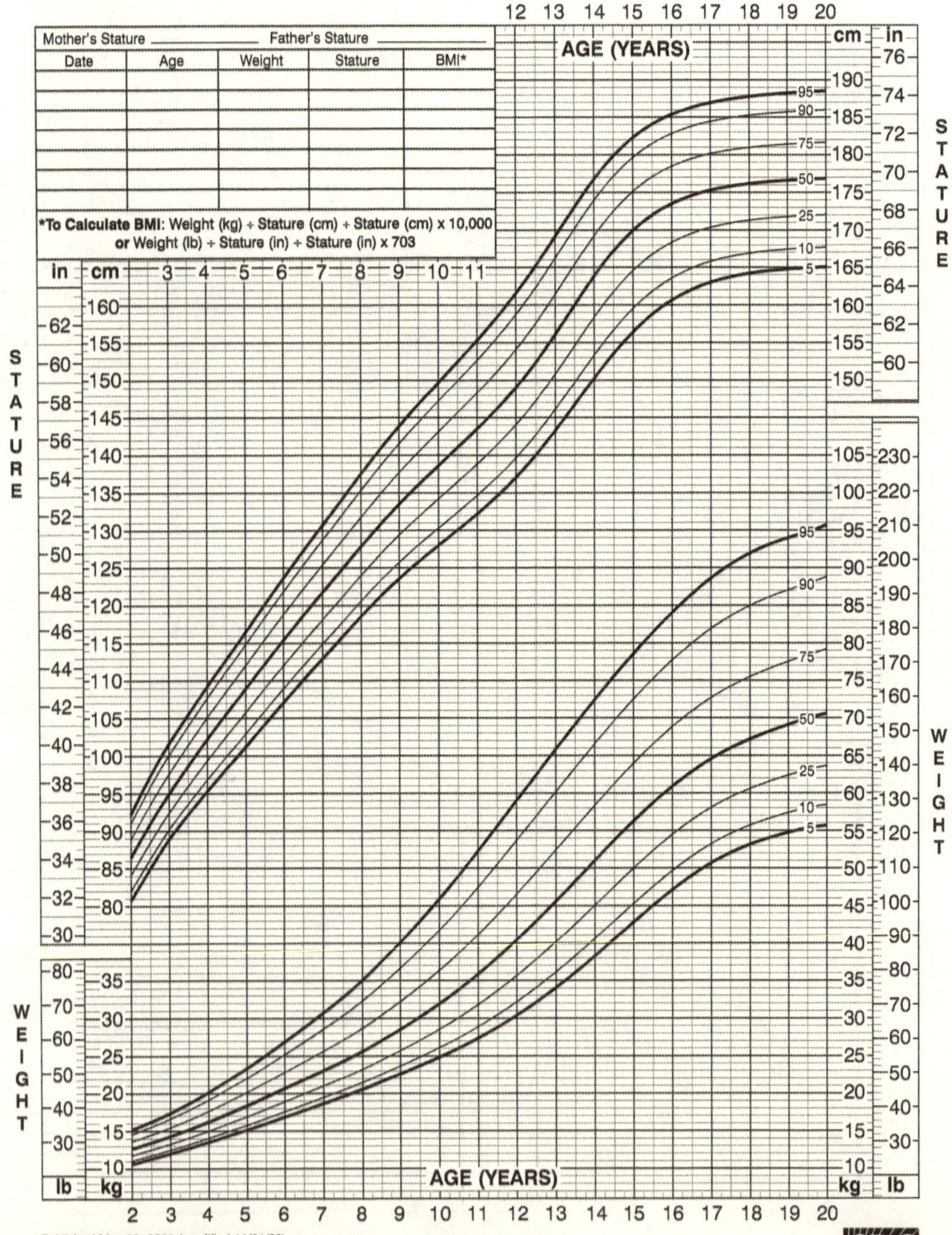

Mother's Stature		Father's Stature		
Date	Age	Weight	Stature	BMI*

*To Calculate BMI: Weight (kg) ÷ Stature (cm) ÷ Stature (cm) x 10,000
or Weight (lb) ÷ Stature (in) ÷ Stature (in) x 703

AGE (YEARS)

12 13 14 15 16 17 18 19 20

STATURE

WEIGHT

cm   in
— 76
190 — 74
185 — 72
180 — 70
175
170 — 68
— 66
165 — 64
— 62
160
155 — 60

95
90
75
50
25
10
5

in cm   3   4   5   6   7   8   9 10 11

in cm
—62—160
—60—155
—58—150
—56—145
—54—140
—52—135
—50—130
—48—125
—46—120
—44—115
—42—110
—40—105
—38—100
—36—95
—34—90
—34—85
—32—80
—30

—80—35
—70—30
—60—25
—50
—40—20
—15
—30
—10

lb kg

STATURE

WEIGHT

AGE (YEARS)

2 3 4 5 6 7 8 9 10 11 12 13 14 15 16 17 18 19 20

cm
105 —230
100 —220
95 —210
90 —200
85 —190
80 —180
75 —170
70 —160
—150
65 —140
60 —130
55 —120
50 —110
45 —100
40 —90
35 —80
30 —70
—60
25 —50
20 —40
15 —30
10

95
90
75
50
25
10
5

kg lb

Published May 30, 2000 (modified 11/21/00)..
SOURCE: Developed by the National Center for Health Statistics in collaboration with
the National Center for Chronic Disease Prevention and Health Promotion (2000).
http://www.cdc.gov/growthcharts

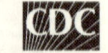

SAFER · HEALTHIER · PEOPLE™

2 to 20 years: Girls
Stature-for-age and Weight-for-age percentiles

NAME _____

RECORD # _____

AGE (YEARS)

Mother's Stature _____		Father's Stature _____		
Date	Age	Weight	Stature	BMI*

*To Calculate BMI: Weight (kg) ÷ Stature (cm) ÷ Stature (cm) x 10,000
or Weight (lb) ÷ Stature (in) ÷ Stature (in) x 703

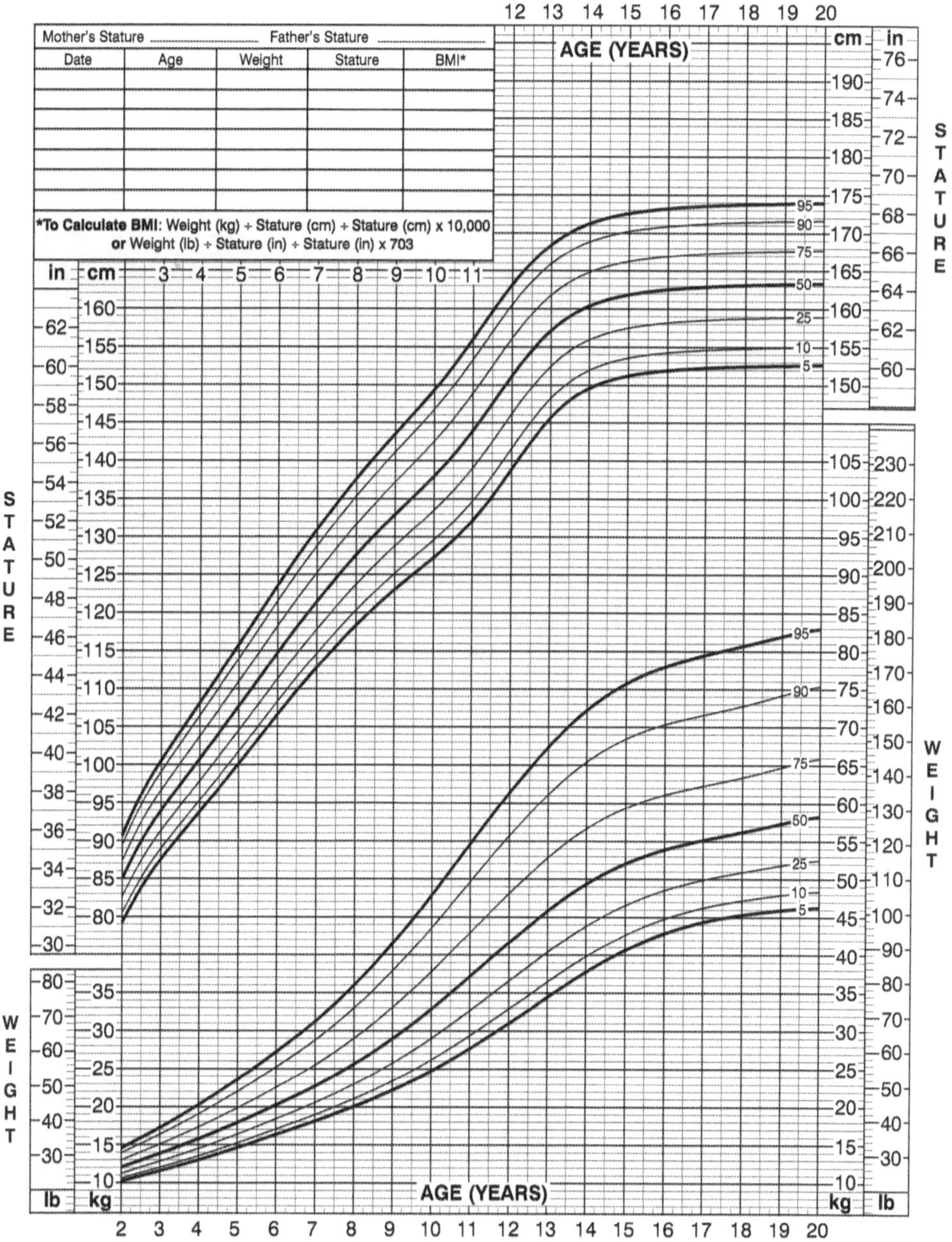

STATURE

WEIGHT

AGE (YEARS)

Published May 30, 2000 (modified 11/21/00).

SOURCE: Developed by the National Center for Health Statistics in collaboration with
the National Center for Chronic Disease Prevention and Health Promotion (2000).
http://www.cdc.gov/growthcharts

SAFER·HEALTHIER·PEOPLE™

2 to 20 years: Boys
Body mass index-for-age percentiles

NAME _____

RECORD # _____

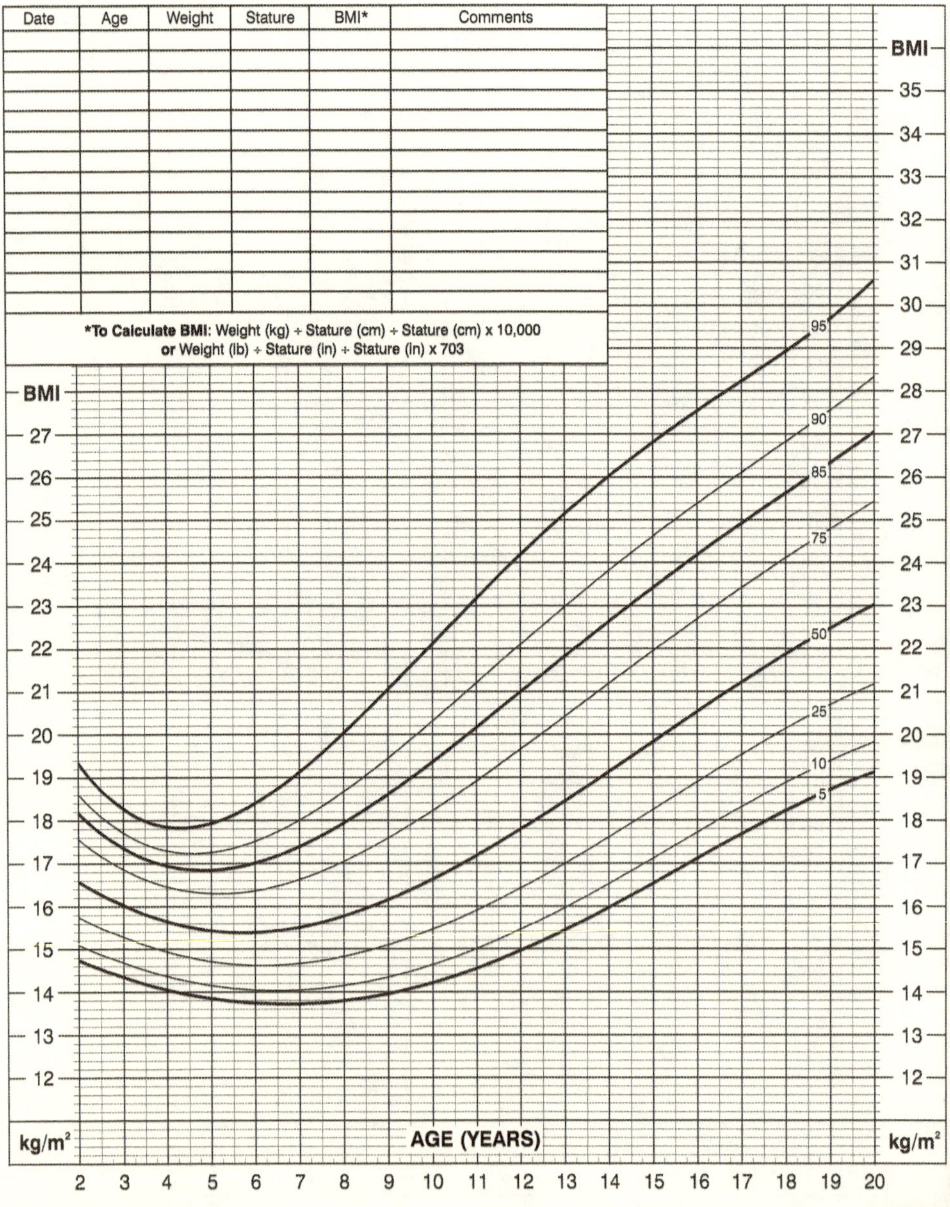

Date	Age	Weight	Stature	BMI*	Comments

*To Calculate BMI: Weight (kg) ÷ Stature (cm) ÷ Stature (cm) x 10,000
or Weight (lb) ÷ Stature (in) ÷ Stature (in) x 703

BMI

35
34
33
32
31
30
29
28
27
26
25
24
23
22
21
20
19
18
17
16
15
14
13
12

BMI

27
26
25
24
23
22
21
20
19
18
17
16
15
14
13
12

95
90
85
75
50
25
10
5

kg/m²

AGE (YEARS)

kg/m²

2 3 4 5 6 7 8 9 10 11 12 13 14 15 16 17 18 19 20

Published May 30, 2000 (modified 10/16/00).
SOURCE: Developed by the National Center for Health Statistics in collaboration with
the National Center for Chronic Disease Prevention and Health Promotion (2000).
http://www.cdc.gov/growthcharts

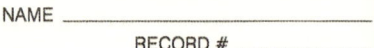

CDC

SAFER · HEALTHIER · PEOPLE™

2 to 20 years: Girls
Body mass index-for-age percentiles

NAME _____

RECORD # _____

Date	Age	Weight	Stature	BMI*	Comments

*To Calculate BMI: Weight (kg) ÷ Stature (cm) ÷ Stature (cm) x 10,000
or Weight (lb) ÷ Stature (in) ÷ Stature (in) x 703

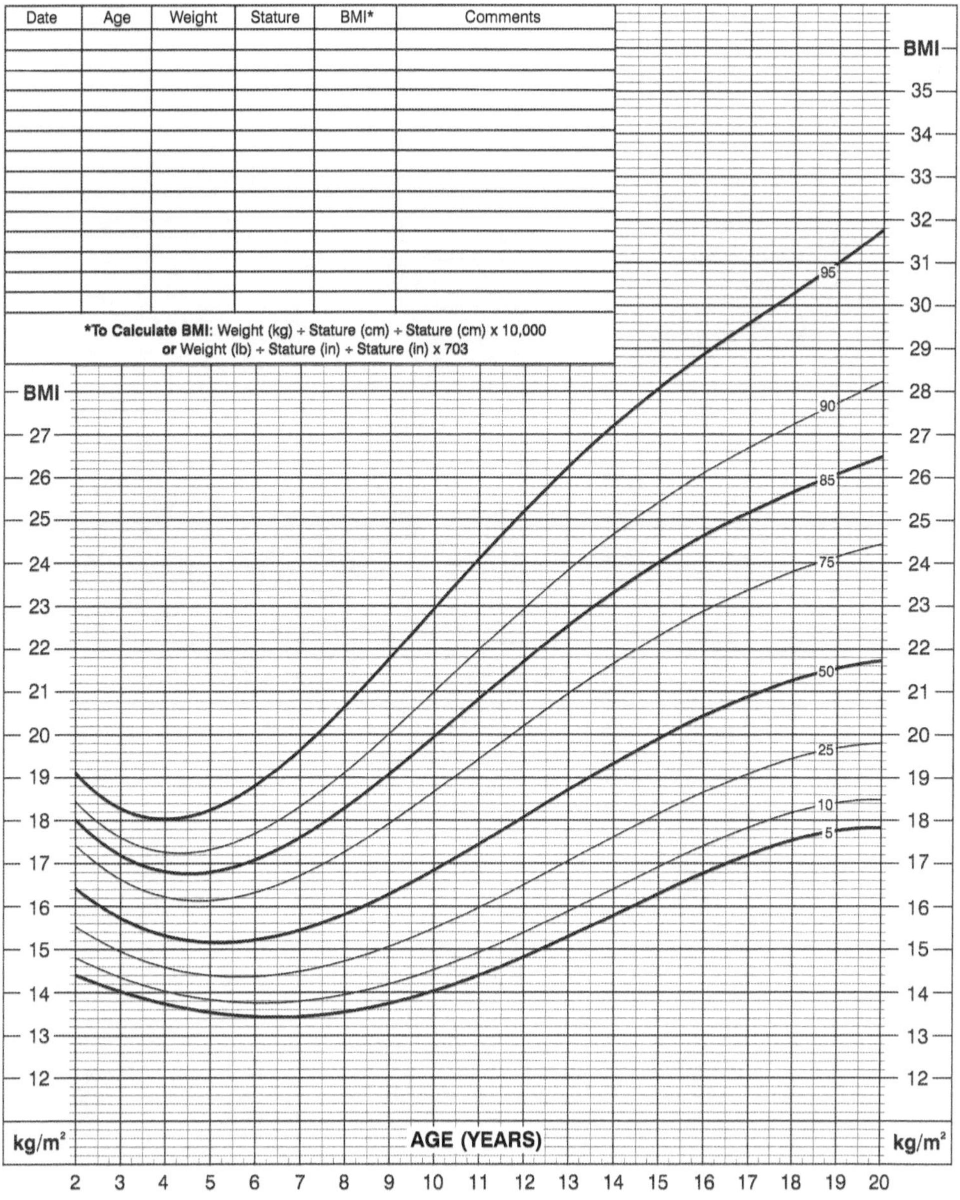

BMI

35
34
33
32
31 — 95
30
29
28 — 90
27
26 — 85
25
24 — 75
23
22
21 — 50
20
19
18 — 25
17 — 10
16 — 5
15
14
13
12

BMI

27
26
25
24
23
22
21
20
19
18
17
16
15
14
13
12

kg/m²   AGE (YEARS)   kg/m²

2 3 4 5 6 7 8 9 10 11 12 13 14 15 16 17 18 19 20

Published May 30, 2000 (modified 10/16/00).
SOURCE: Developed by the National Center for Health Statistics in collaboration with
the National Center for Chronic Disease Prevention and Health Promotion (2000).
http://www.cdc.gov/growthcharts

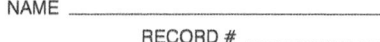

SAFER·HEALTHIER·PEOPLE™

NAME ____________________

Weight-for-stature percentiles: Boys

RECORD # ____________

Date	Age	Weight	Stature	Comments

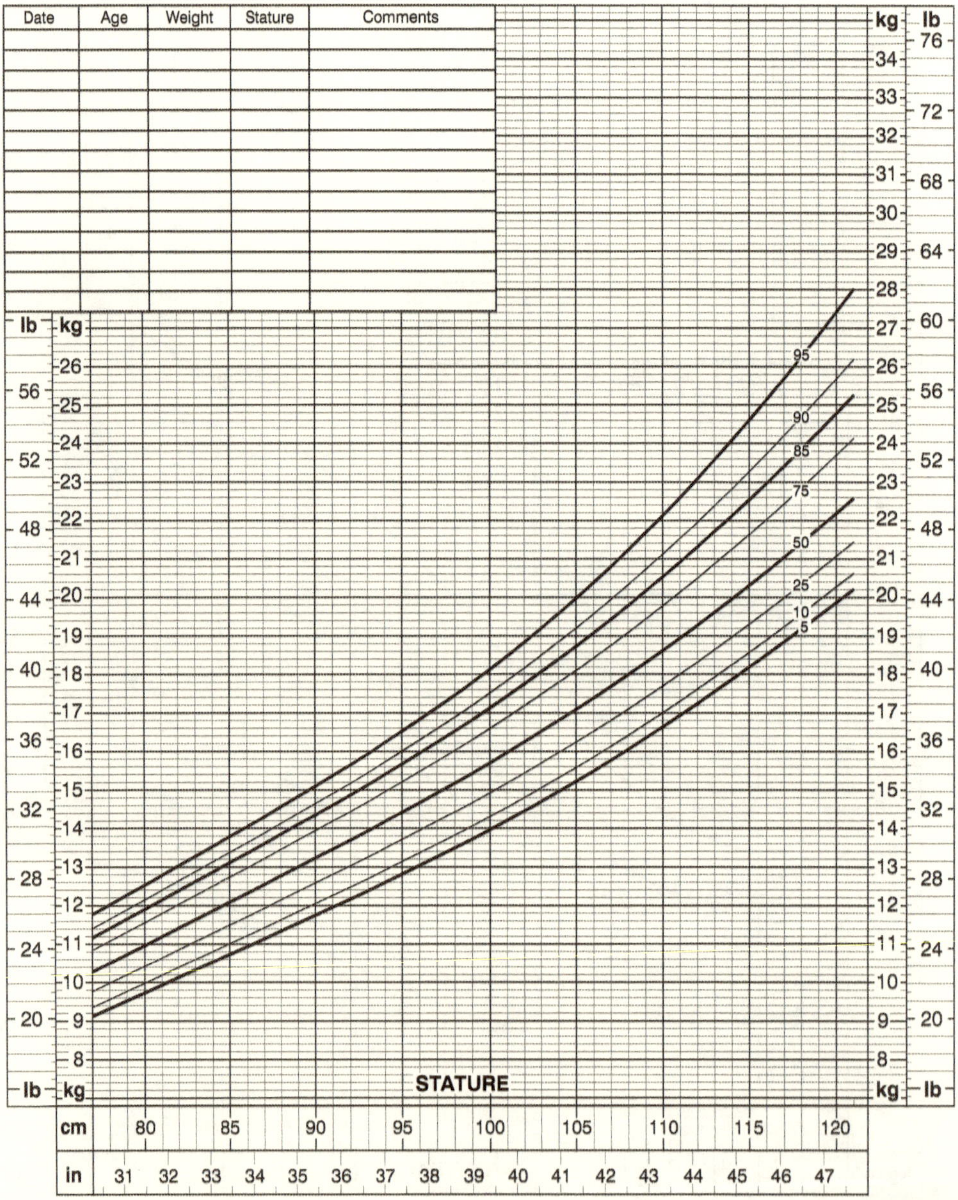

kg
lb
34
33
32
31
30
29
28
27
26
25
24
23
22
21
20
19
18
17
16
15
14
13
12
11
10
9
8
76
72
68
64
60
56
52
48
44
40
36
32
28
24
20
95
90
85
75
50
25
10
5
STATURE
cm
80
85
90
95
100
105
110
115
120
in
31
32
33
34
35
36
37
38
39
40
41
42
43
44
45
46
47

Published May 30, 2000 (modified 10/16/00).
SOURCE: Developed by the National Center for Health Statistics in collaboration with the National Center for Chronic Disease Prevention and Health Promotion (2000).
http://www.cdc.gov/growthcharts

CDC
SAFER • HEALTHIER • PEOPLE™

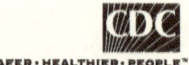

Weight-for-stature percentiles: Girls

Date	Age	Weight	Stature	Comments

STATURE

cm	80	85	90	95	100	105	110	115	120

| in | 31 | 32 | 33 | 34 | 35 | 36 | 37 | 38 | 39 | 40 | 41 | 42 | 43 | 44 | 45 | 46 | 47 |

Percentile curves labeled: 95, 90, 85, 75, 50, 25, 10, 5

Published May 30, 2000 (modified 10/16/00).
SOURCE: Developed by the National Center for Health Statistics in collaboration with
the National Center for Chronic Disease Prevention and Health Promotion (2000).
http://www.cdc.gov/growthcharts

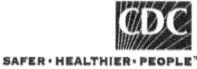

SAFER · HEALTHIER · PEOPLE™

References

1. Berry, D., Sheehan, R., Heschel, R., Knafl, K., Melkus, G. & Grey, M. (2004). Family-based interventions for childhood obesity: A review. *Journal of Family Nursing, 10 (4)*, 249-449.

2. Baughcum, A.E, Chamberlin, L.A. et al., (2000). Maternal perception of overweight preschool children. *Pediatrics, 6:* 1380-1386.

3. Birch, L.L. & Fisher, J.O. (1998). Development of eating behaviors among children and adolescents. *Pediatrics, 101:*593-549.

4. Boyington, J.A. & Johnson, A.A. (2004). Maternal perception of body size as a determinant of infant adiposity in an African-American community. *Journal of the National Medical Association, 96 (3)*, 351-362.

References

5. Calfas, K.J., Zabinski, M.F., & Rupp, J. (2000). Practical nutrition assessment in primary care settings. *American Journal of Preventive Medicine, 18 (14),* 289-299.

6. Casey, R. & Rozin, P. (1989). Changing children's food preferences: Parent opinions. *Appetite, 12:* 171-182.

7. Chen, J.L. & Kennedy, C. (2004). Family functioning, parenting style, Chinese children's weight status. *Journal of Family Nursing, 10 (2),* 262-279.

8. Contento, I.R., Rendell, J.S. & Basch, C.E. (2002). Review and analysis of the evaluation measures used in nutrition education intervention research. *Society for Nutrition Education, 34 (1)* 2-17.

9. Faith, M.S., Berkowitz, R.I., Stallings, V.A., et al. (2004). Parental feeding attitudes and styles and body mass index: Prospective analysis of a gene-environment interaction. *Pediatrics.* Retrieved on December 17, 2004 from http://pediatrics.aappublications.org.

References

10. Fisher, J.O. & Birch, L.L. (1999). Restricting access to palatable foods affect children's behavior, response, food selection, and intake. *The American Journal of Medical Nutrition.* Retrieved on September 16, 2004 from: http://www.ajcn.org.

11. Field, A.E., Colditz, G.A., Fox, M.K., Byers, T., Serdula, M. Bosch, R.J., Peterson, K.E. (1998). Comparison of four questionnaires for assessment of fruit and vegetable intake. *American Journal of Public Health, 88 (8),* 1216-1218.

12. Goodman, E., Hinden, B.R., Khandelwal, S. (2000). Accuracy of teen and parental reports of obesity and body mass index. Retrieved on November 24, 2004 from http://www.findarticles.com.

13. Hammond, K. (2001). Overweight children: Is parental nutrition knowledge a factor? *Food Review, 24 (2),* 18-22.

14. Hardus, P.M., Van Vuuren, C.L., et al. (2003). Public perceptions of the causes and prevention of obesity among

References

primary school children. *International Journal of Obesity, 27,* 1465-1471.

15. Huitt, W., & Hummel, J. (2003). Piaget's theory of cognitive development. *Educational Psychology Interactive.* Valdosta, GA: Valdosta State University. Retrieved January 29, 2004 from: http://chiron.valdosta.edu/whuitt/col/cogsys/piaget.html.

16. Hodges, E. (2003). A primer on early childhood obesity and parental influence. *Pediatric Nursing.* Retrieved on September 29, 2004 from http://www.habermas.org/obesity

17. Jain, A., Sherman, S.N., Chamberlin, L.A., et al. (2001). Why don't low-income mothers worry about their preschoolers being overweight? *Pediatrics, 107 (5),* 1138-1146.

18. Kolody, B. & Sallis, J.F., (1995). A prospective study of ponderosity, body image, self-concept, and psychological variables in children. *Journal of Development & Behavioral Pediatrics, 16:* 1-5.

References

19. Levy, L., Patterson, R.E., et al. (2000). How well do consumers understand percentage daily value on food labels? *American Journal on Health Promotion, 14 (3),* 157-160.

20. Lyle, L.A., Seifert, S., Greenstein, J. & McGovern, P. (2000). How do children's eating patterns and food choices change overtime? Results from a cohort study. *American Journal of Health Promotion, 14 (4),* 222-228.

21. McGraw, S.A., Sellers, D., Stone, E. et al., (2000). Measuring implementation of school programs and policies to promote healthy eating and physical activity among youth. *Preventive Medicine, 31,* S.86-97.

22. McPherson, R.S., Hoelscher, D.M., Alexander, M., et al. (2000). Dietary assessment methods among school age children: Validity and reliability. *Preventive Medicine, 31,* S.11-33.
Mendlein, J.M., Baranowski, T., Pratt, M. (2000). Physical activity and nutrition in children and youth: opportunities for performing

assessments and conducting interventions. *Preventive Medicine,*
31, S.150-153.

23. Mendlein, J.M., Baranowski, T., Pratt, M. (2000). Physical
activity and nutrition in children and youth: opportunities for
performing assessments and conducting interventions. *Preventive*
Medicine, 31, S.150-153.

24. Piper, D.L., Moberg, D.P., King, M.J. (2000). The healthy for
life project: Behavioral outcomes. *The Journal of Primary*
Prevention, 21 (1), 47-73.

25. Puska, P., Nishida, C., & Porter, D. (2003). *Obesity and*
overweight. World Health Organization. Retrieved on
November8,2004 from:
http://www.who.int/hpr/NPH/docs/gs.obesity.pdf.

26. Robinson, T.N., Kiernan, M., et al. (2001). Is parental control
over children's eating associated with childhood obesity? Results

from a population based sample of third graders. *Obesity Research, 9 (5)*, 206-212.

27. Rodgers, B.L. & Knafl, K.A. (2001). *Concept development in nursing: Foundation, techniques, and applications* (2nd ed). Philadelphia: Saunders.

28. Rodgers, B.L. (1989). Concept analysis and the development of nursing knowledge: The evolutionary cycle. *Journal of Advanced Nursing, 14:* 330-335.

29. Satter, E.M. (1990). The feeding relationship: problems and interventions. *The Journal of Pediatrics, 99* (4), e1.

30. Satter, E.M. (1996). Internal regulation and the evolution of normal growth as the basis for prevention of obesity in children. *Journal of the American Dietetic Association, 96* (9), 860-864.

References

31. Stettler, N., Zemel, B.M., et al (2001). Infant, weight gain and childhood overweight status: Multicenter cohort study. *Circulation: Journal of he American Heart Association, 104* (17), II-817-II-818.

32. Siegel, R.V. (2000). *Parental perception of their overweight child vs. child's actual body weight.* Unpublished master's paper. Florida International University, Miami, Florida, USA.

33. Strauss, R.S. (2000). Childhood obesity and self-esteem. *Pediatrics, 105 (1).* Retrieved on September 24, 2004 from http://www.pediatrics.org.

34. Stunkard, A. & Kaplan, D. (1977). Eating in public places: A review of reports of the direct observation of eating behaviors. *International Journal of Obesity, 1:* 89-101.

35. Swadener, S.S. (1994). Nutrition education for preschool age children: A review of research. *Nutrition Education for Preschool Age Children.* Retrieved September 29, 2004 from http://nal.usda.gov.

References

36. Tanasescu, M., Ferris, A.M., Himmelgreen, D.A., et al. (2000). Behavioral factors associated with obesity in Puerto Rican children. *American Society for Nutritional Sciences,* 1734-1742.

37. Troiano, R.P. & Flegal, K.M. (1998). Overweight children and adolescents: description, epidemiology, and demographics. *Pediatrics, 101:* 497-504.

38. U.S Department of Health & Human Services – Public Health (2004, January 21). *Progress review: Nutrition & overweight.* Retrieved on December 9, 2004 from: www.healthypeople.gov/data/2010prog/focus19/default.htm.

39. Wadsworth, B.J. *Piaget's Theory of Cognitive Development.* David McKay Company, Inc., New York, 1974.

40. Waxman M, Stunkard AJ. (1980). Caloric intake and expenditure of obese boys. *The Journal of Pediatrics; 98:* 187–93.

References

Other book or journal references used by the author:

Morrison, G. & Hark, L. (Eds.). (1996). *Medical nutrition and disease.* Cambridge: Blackwell Science.

About the Author
RV Siegel

Born in the Philippines, RV Siegel migrated to the USA in 1993 armed only with her education, a strong will to succeed, and $50 in her pocket. All she knew was that there was a job waiting for her, which was as good a reason as any to make the trip.

She is now happily married to Barry D. Siegel. The couple has two children - David and Amanda.

She works as a Professor at South University, School of Nursing, and has practiced as a Pediatric Nurse Practitioner. She specializes in Pediatric Gastroenterology and Nutrition.

RV Siegel loves to write children's books. Her first, published in 2005, is _"A Bee Called Kangaroo."_ It is the first in a series of children's inspirational books as part of the _Starfish on the Shore_ Book Series.

She is a strong advocate for the rights of the vulnerable and underserved population of America, especially homeless children and children with special needs. As testament to this, 100% of the profits of this book will be donated to Stand Up For Kids [www.standupforkids.org].

RV Siegel's Website:

>_http://www.webspawner.com/users/rvsiegel/index.html_
>_http://mystarfishangel.bravehost.com_

Press Release

April 15, 2005

FOR IMMEDIATE RELEASE:

CONTACT:
RV Siegel
Starfish On The Shore
954.614.7097
MyStarfishAngel@aol.com
http://www.webspawner.com/users/rvsiegel/index.html

RV Siegel Releases New printed & e-Book:

EAT! PEOPLE ARE STARVING IN AFRICA!

2005, Boca Raton, FL: Stop Childhood Obesity, NOW! HERE'S WHY... Preventing children and adolescents from being overweight should be a high priority. In 1998, the World Health Organization has identified childhood obesity as a global epidemic [7,25]. Health disparities among the vulnerable (children, elderly, the poor, etc.) and underserved population is still a major worry and childhood obesity is still, unfortunately a concern. Physicians and nurse practitioners frequently encounter overweight children in their medical practices. However it appears that present interventions used have not been successful since related studies indicated that the percentage of overweight children in the population is rising.

In this very personal yet scientifically accurate book, RV Siegel shares with her readers, one child's bad experiences with food. She was herself that child. As a young girl, the author was taught that she always had to eat everything on her plate, even if she was not hungry. "There are children starving in Africa!" her mother would admonish. With a mixture of guilt and fear the child kept eating until eventually she had developed a serious weight problem. That was followed in adolescence by bouts of binging and purging, potentially fatal actions that she took not knowing what else to do. Thankfully, RV Siegel was able to overcome what she came to call her "demon" and go on to live a normal life as an adult. But her own experiences led her to further research and the realization that poor eating habits – often so severe as to be life-threatening – have become an epidemic amongst millions of our children. Citing the latest research, this gripping book paints a starkly realistic portrayal of this grave problem...and what we as parents, educators and society at large can do to solve it!

Born in the Philippines, RV Siegel migrated to the USA in 1993 armed only with her education, a strong will to succeed, and $50 in her pocket. All she knew was that there was a job waiting for her, which was as good a reason as any to make the trip. She is now happily married to Barry. The couple has two children - David and Amanda. She works as a Professor at South University, School of Nursing, and has practiced as a Pediatric Nurse Practitioner. She specializes in Pediatric Gastroenterology and Nutrition and is currently working on her Doctorate in Educational Leadership.

Press Release

RV Siegel conducted a pilot study regarding parental perception on childhood obesity in 2000 and is currently researching more information regarding parental influences on children's nutrition and eating habits.

RV Siegel also loves to write children's books. Her first, published in the spring of 2005, is **"A Bee Called Kangaroo."** It is the first in a series of children's inspirational books as part of the Starfish on the Shore Book Series. She is a strong advocate for the rights of the vulnerable and underserved population of America, especially homeless children and children with special needs. As testament to this, 100% of the profits of this book will be donated to Stand Up For Kids [www.standupforkids.org].

The bottom line: You are not alone. Understanding different possible factors that influence childhood obesity is the first step. I am hoping that our own personal demons do not affect how we feed our children by over-compensating for what we should and should not do (restricting vs. over-indulgence of palatable foods). I do believe that healthy children have their own "on and off" button that determines their own satiety; that we must be able to tune in and be aware of their subtle cues. They may be saying that they are satisfied and full, and yet, we are so occupied with that "one last ounce" left in the bottle or "just two more bites" on your child's plate that we are negating this innate determination of satiety.

RV Siegel's Website:

>http://www.webspawner.com/users/rvsiegel/index.html
>http://mystarfishangel.bravehost.com

# # #

www.ingramcontent.com/pod-product-compliance
Lightning Source LLC
Chambersburg PA
CBHW030341290526
45785CB00004B/1556